Build your best life

PK Silver Forever

Your Parkour Toolkit

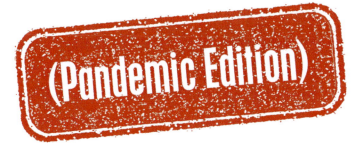

(Pandemic Edition)

Brought to you by the fitness
professionals at PK Move

DISCLAIMER

Please review the following User Agreement carefully before reading/using this book. PK Move strongly recommends that you consult with your physician before beginning any exercise program. You should be in good physical condition and be able to participate in the exercise.

PK Move is not a licensed medical care provider and represents that it has no expertise in diagnosing, examining, or treating medical conditions of any kind, or in determining the effect of any specific exercise on a medical condition.

You should understand that when participating in any exercise or exercise program, there is the possibility of physical injury. If you engage in the exercises described in this booklet or the PK Silver exercise program, you agree that you do so at your own risk, are voluntarily participating in these activities, assume all risk of injury to yourself, and agree to release and discharge PK Move from any and all claims or causes of action, known or unknown, arising out of PK Move's negligence.

IMPORTANT NOTE: Photos in this booklet were taken BEFORE the pandemic and do NOT illustrate proper social distancing. Please maintain 6-10 feet (2-3 meters) between yourself and others at all times. Additionally, the situation caused by COVID-19 may change rapidly from day to day. Always follow directives from your national and local government, health organizations, and of course, your own health care provider.

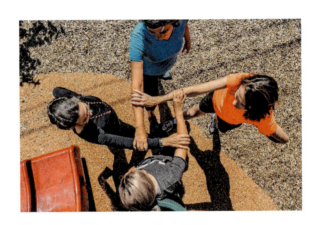

This book is dedicated to our PK Movers.

We would like to thank the entire PK Move Team for their assistance and commitment to our non-profit.

Special gratitude goes out to contributing authors and editors Sean Hannah, Nancy Lorentz, and Angela Hart. Robert Klugerman also contributed many hours to this project as our videographer.

We would also like to express our appreciation to

Eric Rubin

for his belief and support of our mission.

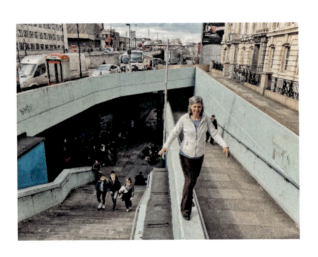

CONTENTS

FOREWORD

Nancy Lorentz,
President and Co-Founder PK Move

PK Move was poised to release our <u>PK Silver Forever: Your Parkour Toolkit</u> when the COVID-19 pandemic was unleashed upon the world. While no one in the world is unaffected, adults who are older or who have underlying medical conditions seem to be at a higher risk should they contract COVID-19. For this reason, they are being urged to stay at home as much as possible. This has led to many questions: How long will this situation last? How do we cope when our normal schedules are completely upended? How can we deal with being physically isolated from our loved ones?

As a result, we decided to modify and add new content to the Toolkit that will be helpful to you during this time. If you are concerned about your wellness, do not despair! You've got this booklet showing steps to refresh or improve your physical activity. Parkour training offers many tools to help you build your best life – even during a pandemic - keeping you independent, strong and capable!

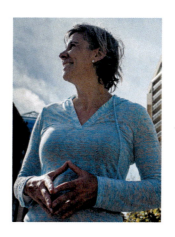

Be strong and be useful,

What is Parkour, PK Move and PK Silver?

Parkour

Parkour is still generally viewed as a daredevil sport for fit, young men performing dangerous stunts in action films! But to truly understand parkour, you must leave Hollywood and travel back in time to 1902 on the island of Martinique, where French Navy Officer George's Hébert was stationed. Hébert arranged the evacuation of hundreds of people when a volcanic eruption took place. He saw his countrymen struggling to move, while the indigenous people easily ran, climbed, and swam away from the disaster to safety. This experience had a great impact on him and would influence his life philosophy and work.

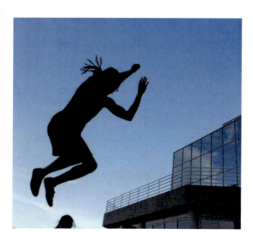

During his naval career, Hébert travelled widely. He was impressed by the physique and movement skills of indigenous peoples in Africa and elsewhere. Later, when he returned to France, he became a physical education pioneer. He developed a training system called "The Natural Method" which revolved around ten basic types of exercise: walking, running, jumping, quadrupedal movement, climbing, balancing, throwing, lifting, self-defense and swimming. He thought these exercises could take place on a spontaneously chosen route or in an obstacle course (le par cours) specifically designed for this purpose.

This obstacle course training was later used by the French military and other emergency workers, such as firefighters. Military obstacle course training became (and still is) the standard for training soldiers, sailors, and emergency responders around the world. In the early 1980s, French Firefighter Raymond Belle instructed his son, David Belle, and a few of his friends in this method of training, "le par cours." It was David Belle who created the word "parkour" and his friends, the Yamakasi, who brought this "new" training discipline into the public eye through documentaries, mind-boggling stunts, commercials, and interviews.

There are many different definitions of parkour, but "using your body to get from Point A to Point B in the fastest, most efficient way possible" is one of the most common.

But parkour is changing. It is emerging as an accessible and beneficial movement practice, even for those who initially would never dream of doing it. At PK Move, we have a different definition:

Parkour is a method of practicing human locomotion.

Critics understandably express skepticism that parkour should be practiced by older adults who haven't run or jumped in many years. The broad range of dynamic movements seen in YouTube videos are generally not recommended for this demographic - that's where *PK Move* comes in!

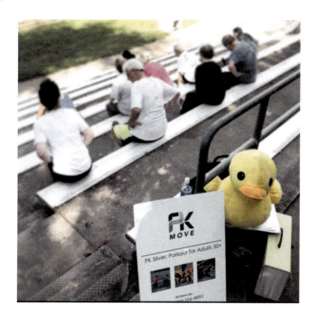

PK Move

PK Move is a non-profit organization founded on the idea that parkour is for everyone. Our mission is to bring the transformative power of parkour to underserved demographics, most notably, older adults. In fact, our flagship program, **PK Silver**, is developed specifically for them! Parkour is a relatively new practice, having been taught professionally in North America for only a little over 15 years. Parkour coaching certifications have matured and expanded to be more inclusive, but still none come close to teaching the proper basics of senior fitness, group fitness, or personal training that are found in nationally recognized senior fitness certifications. If you are lucky enough to find a parkour coach who also holds a nationally recognized fitness certification or degree and is experienced in working with older adults, you are likely in good (and unique) hands, as this is rare.

PK Silver is our answer to the following problems:

- Many senior fitness coaches who hold nationally-recognized certifications or even doctoral degree in physical therapy do not understand or know about parkour.
- Very few parkour coaches have additional certification or education in senior fitness
- Conventional senior fitness training and health models tend to be somewhat rote and favor limiting in the scope of activity in older adults

We wrote **PK Silver Forever: Your Parkour Fitness Toolkit** because of the falls epidemic. That's correct: injuries and complications from falls are the leading cause of accidental death and hospitalization among those 65 years of age and older? Every year, 1 of 4 older adults falls every year, amounting to one fall every second. Now, instead, we are releasing PK Silver Forever: Your Parkour Toolkit, the Pandemic Edition. Although the information we included has been edited and augmented, we want you to remember the falls epidemic has not ceased. Everyone will want to avoid the emergency room and hospitalization as medical teams are stretched very thin caring for COVID-19 patients which are expected to flood our healthcare system. Falls prevention for older adults is more important than ever!

Now let's look back at parkour. What is the main skill that parkour teaches, one that virtually no other practice does?

Parkour teaches how to land safely.

What put parkour on the map was not just that people were jumping between buildings or doing flips outside, it was the fact they could do this in the unforgiving urban environment, without mats, yet not be dashed to pieces. The skills and conditioning techniques developed from parkour training make it unique. Parkour is an art form that doesn't just anticipate the inevitability of falling but uses it to create movements the modern world hasn't seen before. Is there usefulness in this principle that applies to those most vulnerable to falling? Of course! And that's why we developed **PK Silver**.

Let us show you how easy it is to integrate exercise into your life and convince you that **PK Silver, our special brand of parkour for adults 50+,** is an attainable and beneficial component of senior fitness.

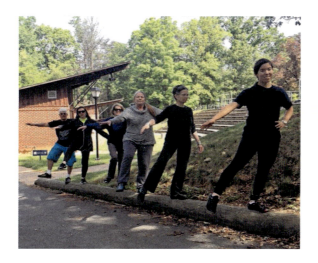

PK Silver

PK Silver helps to prevent falls, enhances health, and enriches your relationship to the world around you even as we struggle with social distancing and other measures taken to battle COVID-19. Let's restart your movement journey so you can emerge from this pandemic stronger than before it started!

Your Fitness: Home, Class, & Community

Assembling spaces in your life for movement is the first step to improving and maintaining your fitness. Where you workout influences the kind of movements you'll do and the opportunities you'll create to connect with others. **PK Move promotes developing at least three spaces for movement in your life - at home, in class, and in the community.**

At Home

During the COVID-19 pandemic, with recommendations that older adults remain at home, this exercise space is most important. You're going to be there more than anywhere else, and sometimes the weather decides getting outside is inaccessible. With dedicated space for movement at home you can always exercise and play, no matter what's going on outside. This is where parkour's playfulness and creativity come in handy! The **PK Silver** curriculum shows you how the simplest home objects - walls, tables, counters, and simple open space - can be used as equipment for building strength, playing games, and learning fall prevention. Hang out with us and pretty soon everything will look like a jungle gym! First, we have to prepare your home for fitness activities. Let's review some simple steps to get you started.

Making Your Home Safe

Now that you are spending more time at home, you can focus on making it safe. We aren't talking about an expensive remodel! There is never a good time to fall, but now, with the medical system under duress, it's imperative to do everything possible to stay injury free.

Here's your pandemic "to do" list. These are simple things that will make your living space healthier and more fall proof.

Keeping it Clean. The Life-Changing Magic of Tidying Up (a popular book by Marie Kondo) could be called The Life-*Saving* Magic of Tidying Up as it applies to falls prevention and good health. That's right, the simple act of cleaning and de-cluttering your home could save your life. **Remove all clutter**, such as stacks of old newspapers and magazines, especially from hallways and staircases to prevent falls. Don't forget to clean your outdoor spaces too. Stair and stairwells as well as decks and patios must be free of clutter and natural debris like sticks and leaves. Once you've tidied up, be sure to **clean and disinfect your home**. While you can't control every germ in your environment, it makes good sense to defend against the germs that can make you sick. The American Cleaning Institute suggests using antibacterial wipes frequently on common-touch surfaces, like the television remote, faucet handles, doorknobs and light switches.

Repair or remove hazards. Now that your home is clean, take time to cast a critical eye over every room, hall, and stairway. Look for hazards such as loose carpet, slippery throw rugs, floorboards or nails that stick up. Don't forget look for hazards on outdoor stairs, decks, and patios. This includes rickety furniture. Repair, remove, or replace any hazardous items you find. Additionally, you should add non-slip mats or carpets in areas that can become slipper, like the bathroom or kitchen.

Let the Light Shine In. Does your home have adequate lighting? If not, add some brighter light bulbs. Call a relative or handyman to install more lights or brighter light bulbs where needed, especially in stairways and hallways, both inside and outside your home. Purchase a few night-lights for bedrooms and bathrooms to make it easier to see at night.

Rails and bars. It's a sad, but common occurrence that many people fix their loose railings or install grab bars AFTER a fall occurs. Obviously, this is the wrong order! When you call your relative or handyman about installing new or more powerful lighting, ask to have your loose rails (indoors and outdoors) repaired or installed and grab bars installed in the bathroom. While these items can prevent falls, we often use them to perform fun exercises in **PK Silver**!

Make Space for Exercise

Once you've finished tidying, cleaning, and repairing your home, it's time to prepare your exercise space. You may have a room that can be dedicated to exercise, but that's not necessary. You can use a room that has multiple purposes, like a living room which may be where you entertain guests, watch TV, and read. All that is needed is:

Space. In most living rooms, there is a coffee table or ottoman in the middle of the space. Simply move this out of the way!

Large Rug. Hopefully you already have a rug in the room, or it is carpeted.

Other items which are *nice* to have, but NOT necessary are a large mirror (to check your form), a radio or blue tooth speaker for music, a basket for your yoga mat, a towel, maybe some dumbbells or bands. If you are following workouts on TV, you'll need a TV in the room. If you're watching videos or live-stream workouts, you'll need a smart phone, laptop or computer.

Get Out

Now you have everything you need to begin exercising inside, but there is a reason we wanted you to repair hazards, check lighting, and clean *outside* too. Now you have multiple places to work out at home! **PK Silver** is practiced outside whenever possible. Did you know that research suggests that outdoor exercise might have even more health benefits than the gym? Since the gym is closed anyway, let's look at why exercising outdoors is particularly important during this stressful pandemic when we are all also combatting cabin fever.

> While outdoors on a sunny day, you receive a dose of Vitamin D
>
> Outdoor activities through green space lower stress
>
> Outdoor exercise is associated with greater decreases in tension, confusion, anger and depression when compared to indoor activity
>
> Just five minutes of exercise in a "green space" such as a park can boost mental health

In Class

Your next movement space would normally be a fitness class. At this time, we do not recommend joining any in-person classes, BUT thanks to the internet, there are many options available to live-stream classes right into your home. There are SO many benefits to attending classes such as learning new skills, reviving old ones, working out harder than you would alone, and cultivating a source of FUN in your life!

The Baby Boomer population has fueled an explosion in the number of senior-oriented fitness classes, such as **PK Silver**. Do a little research, find a class, and sign up! Fitness classes are obviously good for exercise and everything else we mentioned, but their greatest value lies in the opportunity to meet people and build relationships – even virtual relationships - that will help you stay motivated. Check our website (www.pkmove.org) to sign up for live, on-line **PK Silver** classes, as well as videos.

Another option is dusting off the VCR and popping in that Jane Fonda aerobics tape from the 80s! Got rid of all those old tapes? Her videos and many others are available on YouTube. A few other tips for on-line or video classes:

- Be sure your exercise space is tidy and ready with all the equipment you'll need for class. Especially if you're a beginner, be sure someone is at home with you during the class
- Wear athletic closed-toe shoes with a closed heel and clothing that is comfortable to move in, but not too loose. Avoid pants or skirts that drag on the ground. Avoid shoes such as Crocs or sandals.

In the Community

This is a tough time for the community aspect with many saying we are "alone together." You are supposed to stay at home as much as possible, but as mentioned earlier, that doesn't mean you can't go outside . . . just maintain a safe distance of 6-10 feet (2-3 meters) between yourself and others. You may be able to speak with neighbors or say "hello" to passers-by. It is vital for your health and well-being to creating space for movement that allows for some kind of social interaction when you go outside to play!

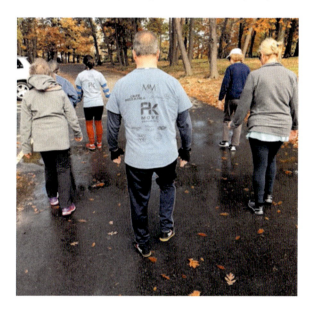

If you are concerned about going to a park, bring a person from your household and go earlier in the day, before most people are out. If you are older and have underlying health conditions, you can stick to walking in your neighborhood. You can walk up and down your driveway, or (if you're lucky to either available) use your garden or green space around your home or apartment.

Enjoying life and spending time with our loved ones is more important than ever right now. We suggest that you:

Plan regular walks with a member of your household. If you live alone, ask a family member or close friend to join you.

Set up regular phone calls or video chats with friends and family. There are many ways to do video chats, such as by FaceTime or Zoom. Ask for help if needed.

Limit screen time. Our on-line lives are now in overdrive. We urge you to take short breaks, every hour, to move around and preferably go outside. Only five minutes outdoors can make a major difference in your mindset. While you want to stay current with the news during this global health emergency, be careful to limit news intake; the news cycle can create a lot of stress. If you are feeling stressed, call a family member or friend to talk about it, go for a walk or take some deep breaths. (A calming breath video is included with the **PK Silver** Daily 5 videos.)

WHEN EXERCISING IN PUBLIC SPACES DURING THE PANDEMIC

If there are more than a handful of people in the green space, do NOT enter the area. Choose a different area or return home.

Stay informed and always follow local guidance for the latest health recommendations with regard to usage of public parks and other public spaces.

Consistently & Persistently

Once you have spaces in your life for movement, you must use them! Health through movement is a lifetime pursuit, and none of us gets it perfectly, but where there is consistency - if goals are set, more or less met, and then reset - progress always comes. Ideally, we could just play randomly, as children do. But we're not children, so we must take play a bit seriously. Grownup tools like planning, scheduling, and accountability still have their place and enable us to make the most of playtime!

Planning.

Constantly ask yourself "What are my goals and how do I achieve them?" Without a clear vision of the movements you desire most - "I want to pick up my grandkids," "I want to go up and down stairs comfortably," "I want to go to Italy and walk the cobblestone streets without pain," etc. - your training will be unfocused and inconsistent. PK Move recommends having three specific movement goals to work on at any one time. Plan your workouts accordingly so that your goals determine the workout you select.

For example, if "picking up my granddaughter" were the goal, first visualize that movement in its optimum form - a low, steady squat with a strong, straight back supplying a base, using the arms to grab and hold a weight between 10 and 50 lbs., and then standing with the weight using proper form, free of pain.

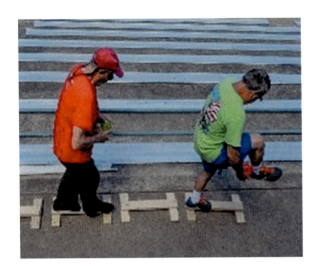

Exercise is not terribly complicated once you know what you want to do. This is another reason the movement-based approach of **PK Silver** is so different - "being fit" is too vague to be meaningful. We must first SEE IN OUR MIND the movements that have meaning, and then bring them to life. We'd love to show you how!

Scheduling.

Once you know what your goals are, make time for them. This is why we like classes - it makes planning easier. Whatever goals you have will take priority in the exercise classes you select. For instance, if you want to carry your groceries with strength and good balance, you will sign up for a **PK Silver** class. After that, it's just planning around the class. For example, if you were taking **PK Silver** on a certain day, that would be the "start of your movement week" and the schedule fills out from there. Take the next day to recover with light exercise. The next day is another class or group event specific to achieve a goal, like dancing or hiking. Take another recovery day with healing work like stretches or massage. The next day go to a park to work on your **PK Silver** skills with a friend. The next day is a long walk around a park, etc. Ta-da! We now have a schedule:

Day 1: PK Silver
Day 2: Recovery plus 30 minutes walking
Day 3: Goal-specific class
Day 4: Recovery plus stretching
Day 5: Park day with friend(s)!
Day 6: Long walk (45-60 minutes)
Day 7: Recovery

See? Just like that, you have planned a whole week of movement. Look at you go!

Staying on track

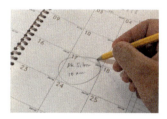

Plans and schedules are great, but for any of it to work you must be accountable. To us, accountability is all about "The Three Fs" - ***Firmness, Forgiveness, Friendship.***

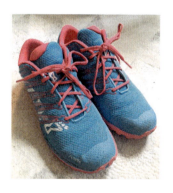

Firmness.

It's just another way to say "prioritize!" Once you've made a plan to move and you have a schedule, that's it. Let nothing stop you! We're all good at justifying inconsistency - social opportunities, lack of sleep, a new TV show, forgetfulness, etc. The reasons we come up with to neglect movement just multiply if we're not resolved to make it a central part of our life. If it really matters, Be Firm about it.

Forgiveness.

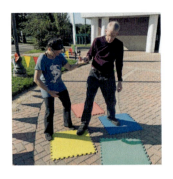

Now, let's be clear – as firm as you may be, there's a chance you're going to mess up from time to time. It happens, especially during a pandemic! Fitness is forever challenging, and some days we just don't have the motivation or time in our schedule. Beating yourself up doesn't help. It pushes you the wrong direction - away from movement. Instead, create the space within yourself to say "I failed today, and that's ok. I might fail again tomorrow, and that's ok too. I'm going to try anyways." This attitude of forgiveness is the bedrock of persistence, which keeps you going on the days when you don't feel like it, and better able to see the small bits of progress that still happen anyways. Best of all, when forgiveness becomes a healthy habit you stop caring about progress and just have fun when you move, which makes progress come quicker.

Friendship.

This is extremely important during the pandemic. Of the many benefits working out with friends offers, accountability to each other is perhaps the most valuable. We can let ourselves down easier than we can let someone else down, which makes "the buddy system" of working out so effective. Create a culture of movement in your relationships and you'll have a bottomless well of support. Plus, if your friends are willing to explore new online classes and walk the neighborhood with you, your workouts become adventures. Now you have a pandemic story! Who would cancel on that?

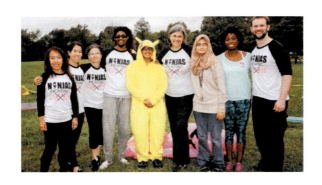

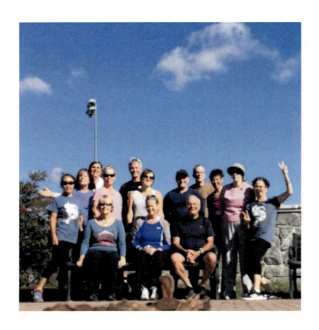

Coaching Excellence

A fitness class, even an online fitness class, is an integral part of your movement journey. Nobody does this all by themselves. Having reliable, knowledgeable coaches that you connect with makes the journey more productive and fun. So, how does one find great teachers? Many people just follow the recommendations of their friends. We have some further suggestions. Knowing your goals should come before anything else. Once your goals are set, look for a class. When you find a class you're interested in, seek information about the instructor. You may be able to simply watch some previews of the class and see if you like their coaching style, but we recommend contacting them first and asking some pertinent questions:

> **How long have they been teaching?**

> **What's their experience in senior fitness? Do they have certifications?**

> **How big is the class? Can they give you individual attention? Is there more than one instructor on hand?**

Ideally, your instructor will have some experience working with seniors, either directly in their classes or in some other aspect of their profession (physical therapy, etc.). If they don't, but you still want to take the class, it's important to find out if they have **CPR/First Aid/AED training.** Even though they are currently teaching on-line, as a fitness professional they should have their CPR/First Aid at a minimum to recognize if you are having any adverse health conditions during class.

PK Silver has the following requirements:

PK Silver Coaches are trained in our program *plus*

hold valid First Aid/CPR certificate
pass background check
Have additional senior fitness training, university degrees, or national certification such as ACSM, NASM, ACE, AAFA, etc.

PK Silver Classes are capped at 15 participants with 2 coaches.
Average class size is 10 participants

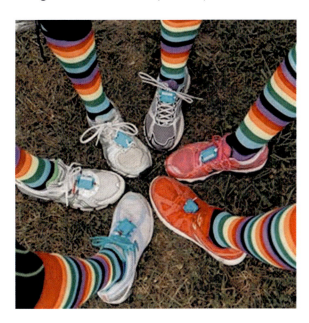

Equipment & Clothing

Right now, no one is going to the gym. If for some unexpected reason a gym is open in your community during the coronavirus pandemic, we highly recommend you avoid it since gyms are high-transmission locations. Even **PK Silver** classes, which normally **come to YOU,** have been suspended at this time. We have decided to offer **PK Silver** exercise videos online and via virtual coaching sessions to help battle inactivity during the pandemic. We will come back to your senior community center, your house of worship, or your neighborhood park when the pandemic is under control and public health officials say it is safe to do so.

You may notice that other fitness programs sell special equipment to use at home. To be clear, we are NOT against those things, but our program is completely different. **PK Silver** requires very little, if any equipment. We pride ourselves on being able to offer a fun, challenging workout even in an empty room or open field. We mostly rely on curbs, railings, steps, trees, picnic tables (outside) or furniture, steps, rails, kitchen counters, and other everyday objects as obstacles.

If you want to come to a **PK Silver** online or in person class, what should you do? What should you bring or wear?

Read and complete all required forms and waivers

Wear clothes which are comfortable for moving around and are appropriate for the current weather.

Wear appropriate closed-toe shoes with an enclosed heel (no sandals, mules, clogs, crocs)

Have drinking water available

Be capable of moving about independently with minimal assistance

Tend to personal needs independently (toilet, medication, etc.)

Sometimes you may be asked to bring a yoga mat or towel

As noted, **PK Silver** athletes do not need special clothing to train parkour. In cold or transitioning weather, please wear layers, such as a jacket or top over a t-shirt, so you can add or peel off clothes as needed to remain happy and healthy.

Fitness Assessment

Before you begin an in-person **PK Silver** class, we will ask you to complete several forms as well as a fitness assessment. Obviously, we cannot perform this assessment now that our locations are shut down. However, if you are taking on-line classes you must complete our online waiver and the PAR-Q which stands for "physical activity readiness questionnaire." If you decide to skip on-line classes for now and decide to stick with the "**PK Silver** Daily 5", we strongly suggest you take a moment to fill out the PAR-Q. If you answer "YES" to one or more questions on the PAR-Q, please call, email, or video chat with your doctor about whether or not you may do the "**PK Silver** Daily 5"

PAR-Q & YOU

Physical Activity Readiness Questionnaire

Regular physical activity is fun and healthy and increasingly more people are starting to become more active everyday. Being more active is very safe for most people. However, some people should check with their doctor before they start becoming much more physically active.

If you are planning to become much more physical active than you are now, start by answering the seven questions in the box below. If you are between ages of 15 and 69, the PAR-Q will tell you if you should check with your doctor before you start. If you are over 69 years of age, and you are not used to being very active, check with your doctor.

Common sense is your best guide when you answer these questions. Please read the questions carefully and answer each one honestly: check YES or NO.

YES	NO	
☐	☐	1. Has you doctor said that you have a heart condition and/or that you should only do physical activity recommended by a doctor?
☐	☐	2. Do you feel pain in your chest when you do physical activity?
☐	☐	3. In the past month, have you had chest pain when you were not doing physical activity?
☐	☐	4. Do you lose you balance because of dizziness or do you ever lose consciousness?
☐	☐	5. Do you have a bone or joint problem (for example, back, knee or hip) that could be made worse by a chance in your physical activity?
☐	☐	6. Is your doctor currently prescribing drugs (for example, water pills) for your blood pressure or heart-condition?
☐	☐	7. Do you know of <u>any other reason</u> why you should not do physical activity?

If you answered

YES to one or more questions

Talk with your doctor by phone or in person BEFORE you start becoming much more physically active or before you have a fitness appraisal. Tell your doctor more about the PAR-Q and which questions you answered yes

NO to all questions

If you answered NO honestly to all PAR-Q questions, you can be reasonably sure that you can:

- Start becoming much more physically active – begin slowly and build up gradually. This is the safest and easiest way to go.
- Take part in a fitness appraisal – this is an excellent way to determine your fitness so that you can plan the best way for you to live actively. It is highly recommended that you have your blood pressure evaluated. If your reading is over 144/94, talk with your doctor before you start becoming much more physically active.

DELAY BECOMING MUCH MORE ACTIVE

- If you are not feeling well because of a temporary illness such as a cold or a fever – wait until you feel better or
- If you are or may be pregnant – talk to your doctor before you start becoming more active

PLEASE NOTE: If your health changes so that you then answer YES to any of the above questions, tell your fitness or health professional. Ask whether you should change your physical activity plan.

Informed Use of the PAR-Q: PK Move Inc., USA Parkour, and their agents assume no liability for persons who undertake physical activity, and if in doubt after completing this questionnaire, consult your doctor prior to physical activity.

NOTE: If the Par-Q is being given to a person before he or she participates in a physical activity program or a fitness appraisal, this section may be used for legal or administrative purposes.

"I have read, understood and completed this questionnaire. Any questions I had were answered to my full satisfaction."

NAME _____

SIGNATURE   DATE

Health is Wealth

The Center for Disease Control states that "older adults and people of any age who have serious underlying medical conditions may be at higher risk for more serious complications from COVID-19." What should you do?

The Big Four

Face Mask Advice on face masks has changed a lot since March 2020 and it may change again after we publish this eBook. Always follow your local and federal guidelines. PK Move recommends that you cover your mouth and nose with a cloth face cover when

- you have to go out in public, for example to the grocery store or to pick up other necessities, or
- you are around people you don't live with.

Continue to keep about 6 feet between yourself and others. The cloth face cover is not a substitute for social distancing.

Wash Your Hands Wash your hands with soap and water for at least 20 seconds. Then wash them again. And again. And… you get the picture! Seriously, this is an extremely important protective step to keep the virus at bay. Anytime you train parkour, you will be touching some object in or outside your home. Even if you already cleaned that object, assume it is dirty and WASH YOUR HANDS when you are finished training! Be careful not to touch your face between hand washings.

Social Distancing At of the time of publication, the CDC is recommending that older adults and those with underlying health conditions stay home and only go out only for essential food or health needs. When seniors do go out, they must practice social distancing. This means limiting the overall number of contacts you have with others. Every contact is a risk of catching the virus, you need to limit your circle to those in your household. Secondly, it means keeping others, especially visitors (even your adorable grandchildren) at least six feet away. If they can't maintain this distance, they shouldn't be visiting. If you're out for a walk, steer clear of others. If you live alone, it may be nice to contact a relative, close friend, or neighbor to walk with you, but be careful to keep the 6-foot distance.

Clean High-Touch Surfaces Your kitchen counter and table, your TV remote control, your doorknobs - any surface touched by you, those in your home, and those who visit - are considered high-touch surfaces. Clean every day, multiple times per day. If you go out to train parkour in a public park, even if the park is empty, assume all railing, benches, picnic tables, and so forth are dirty. We do not recommend touching any items in the park unless you intend to thoroughly clean them or wear latex gloves. In both cases, take care and test your grip before performing exercises. Dispose of gloves in trash can immediately after use and wash hands. For more information visit www.cdc.gov

Keep Moving!

Regular exercise is absolutely essential during this time. Exercise will help you sleep better and reduce stress. At minimum, do the **PK Silver** Daily 5 every day.

Make an Emergency Plan

At the end of this booklet, we invite you to write down all people in your movement support team. Use that list to make a plan of who you will call when you need help if you're having difficulty meeting basic needs like obtaining food and medicine or taking care of yourself in the event you become sick during the pandemic.

Finally, some hopeful news:

The oldest person to survive the virus is 103-year old Zhang Guangfen. She had no underlying health issues and was released from the hospital after only 6 days. Additionally, a 100-year-old man with heart failure, Alzheimer's and hypertension also recovered from the disease in Wuhan, China after being treated. England's chief medical officer, Chris Whitty, says there's a common misconception that all elderly people who contract the virus die from it:

"I think it's easy to get a perception that if you are older and you get this virus then you're a goner. Absolutely not, the great majority of people will recover from this virus, even if they are in their 80s."

PK Silver Building Blocks

Our approach to movement and fall prevention relies in large part on the existing knowledge of senior fitness gathered by physical therapists, hospitals, and established fall prevention programs. However, what makes **PK Silver** different is our focus on locomotion - the ability to move from one place to another.

This concept of getting from Point A to Point B efficiently and creatively is novel in a world of senior fitness that likes to keep its participants in one spot while performing rote, isolated movements. There is value in this since it helps build a foundation for movement, but it's not the same as locomotion - walking, running, climbing, crawling, swinging . . . the fun stuff! These playful skills are the bedrock of our curriculum, which is why it's so effective and so enjoyable!

You will practice the correct forms of the building blocks of functional fitness. The names of many of these exercises will be familiar to you, such as the lunge, while others, like the QM (which stands for quadrupedal movement) may be new vocabulary. Here are the **PK Silver** Building Block Exercises which you can practice now to keep yourself strong and mobile:

Single-Leg Balance

How to do it: Find a sturdy object, such as the kitchen counter. Start in front of this object while standing in a tall, upright position with feet parallel and hands resting lightly on the counter. Shift weight to right leg. The crown of your head, your right hip, and your right heel should be stacked in a vertical column as you raise left foot slightly off the ground (no more than 1-inch!) Make sure both hips are parallel to and equally distanced from your kitchen counter or supportive object. Avoid leaning into your hip. Now take your fingers off the counter one-by-one, beginning with your pinky finger until only your thumb remains. If your balance feels steady, remove one thumb and then both thumbs, and allow your hands to hover no more than 1-inch about the counter. If you begin to lose balance, simply put your foot down and place hands on the counter, returning to the start position. Work your way up to. Alternate on the other leg. Work your way up to holding your balance for 30 seconds on each leg without needing hands on the counter.

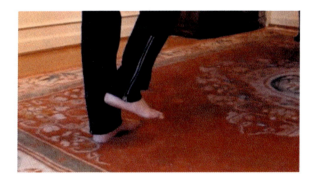

If you are waving your hands around wildly and/or feel yourself pitching, STOP doing this exercise and see your doctor or physical therapist. You need specific exercises to strengthen your balance before attempting this exercise.

Walking

It seems simple, but after living a potentially less active life and aging a few years, many older adults begin to shuffle. Here are our pointers on how to "Walk the Walk." First, *stand up straight* and tall! Pretend someone had grabbed a fistful of your hair (if you have any hair left on your head!) and is pulling you straight up off the ground. Shoulders should be relaxed and let your *arms hang and swing naturally* as you walk. Now start walking! Your pace should be even and steady. Don't take huge steps! *Keep your steps short and comfortably fast.* How fast? Think of the song "Stayin' Alive" by the Bee Gees which is 103 beats per minute (BPM) and results in a 20-minute mile. That's a good pace. If this seems too fast or slow for you, know that the commonly recommend range when selecting music to walk to is 80-140 BPM. AC/DC's "Shook Me All Night Long" is 81 BPM.

However, the most important aspect of walking is heel-to-toe motion or shifting your bodyweight as you walk.

For example, your right heel should be the first part of your foot to touch the ground. Rolling through the ball of the foot, push off with your toes. At the same time that you are pushing off with your right toes, your left heel should be touching the ground. Grab a buddy and try to walk like this for at least 20 minutes per day.

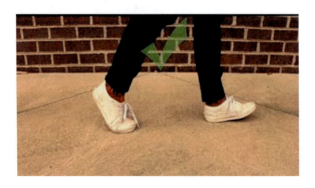

Test your heart rate by seeing if you can talk to your walking buddy. If you can't and/or are struggling for breath, you're going too fast! If you can talk easily, try singing, because if you can sing and walk, you're moving too slowly!

Chair Squat

Stand in front of a sturdy chair as if you are about to sit down. Your feet should be just wider than shoulder width and your toes should point outward. Stand up tall. As you sit down into your squat, lead with your bottom moving toward the back of the chair. Keep your knees out and moving in the direction your toes are pointing. Your back should be kept relatively straight with the abdominal muscles engaged as you maintain good posture. Once seated, your shins should be at the same angle as your back. To get back up, squeeze the glute muscles of the buttocks, stand up tall and straight (do not rock forward) and keep those knees wide. **If you are feeling pain in your knees while doing this exercise, stop immediately!** Pain means your form is not correct and/or you need to do another version of this exercise.

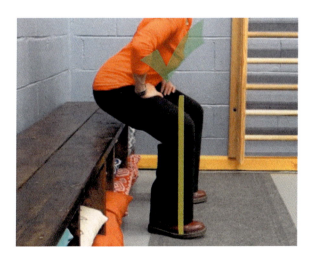

QM Variations

QM stands for *Quadrupedal Movement* and means "moving on four legs." For human development, this is normally limited to babies who crawl. Because we quickly graduate to bipedal movement (walking on two legs), we rarely go back to crawling, but we are going back now to make your core and upper body stronger. If you are not accustomed to getting up and down from the ground, don't worry, we have variations for you. Below is a description of the static QM stance for **PK Silver**. Please come to class or see our website to learn dynamic variations.

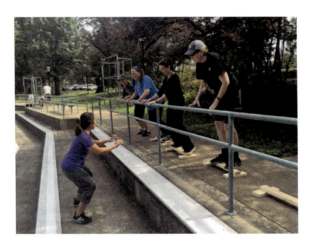

Stand with feet shoulder width apart and about two feet (measure using your own feet) from sturdy railing or countertop, such as kitchen counter. (If this railing is wobbly or the counter is slippery... you know what to do: fix it! Call a handy person to come fix all loose railings and keep surfaces clean.) Place your hands on the rail/counter, also about shoulder width apart. Lower your center of gravity into a shallow squat, no more than 10-20%. Now shift your weight forward toward the rail/counter. You will likely feel your heels come off the ground as you begin to stand on to the balls of your feet and toes. As a result, you take more weight into your arms and shoulders. Be sure your back is straight, not arched, and your tummy is pulled in as if someone were about to tickle you. Slowly absorb more weight with your arms, then push away from the rail/counter and stand up fully. To make this easier, stand closer to the rail/counter. To make it more difficult, stand farther away. **Don't overdo or push through pain.** This is an easy exercise to do at home or at the park on a picnic table or railing. *Again, verify the obstacle is clean and sturdy before touching or putting weight on it.*

Stretches

After a prolonged period of sitting (30 minutes or more) you should get up to move and do some simple stretches.

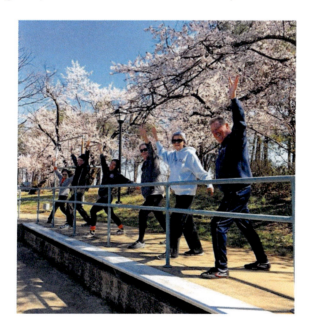

A free video of these stretches are available at **www.pkmove.org.**

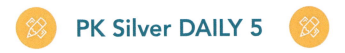

PK Silver DAILY 5

Check with your doctor *before starting any new exercises or fitness programs, especially if you have been sedentary for a period of time.* If you are cleared for take-off, do these exercises daily to improve balance and increase strength.

PK Silver DAILY 5
- ✓ Single-Leg Balance (3 seconds per leg, next to counter)
- ✓ Walk (20 minutes per day)
- ✓ Chair Squats before meals (1-8 squats, 3 times per day
- ✓ QM variations (5 minutes per day)
- ✓ Get up, MOVE, and stretch (5 minutes per hours, minimum)

Check with your doctor before beginning any exercise program
www.pkmove.prg | 571-836-4094 | info@pkmove.org

Free videos of these *FIVE PK Silver* building blocks are available at www.pkmove.org for your convenience.

Your Movement Support Team

Your health is of paramount importance to you, to your family and friends, to your community and, yes, to your nation. We need you! Keeping you moving is a project much bigger than yourself. The happiest, most successful movers have a whole team in their corner. We're not talking about Olympic athletes. *We're talking about YOU.*

Everyone in your life should make a positive contribution to your health, no matter how small. Starting with us, we want you to fill out the rest of this page and realize just how big your team is. These people are resources to help you on your journey, be it through expert advice, direct care, or emotional support.

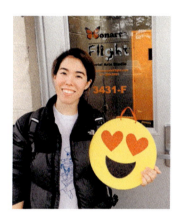

Never forget that your individual fitness is a TEAM SPORT.
The PK Move Team is here to support you!

NAME	TELEPHONE	WEBSITE	STREET ADDRESS
PK Move	571-386-4094	www.pkmove.org	
Family			
Friends			
Neighbors			
Doctor			
Dentist			
Optometrist			
Pharmacy			
Physical Therapist			
Personal trainer			
House of Worship			
IN CASE OF EMERGENCY CALL 911			

CONTACT US

Looking for a PK Silver Coach in your area?

Visit
www.pkmove.org

for details and registration infomation

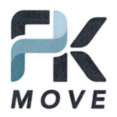

Made in the USA
Las Vegas, NV
03 July 2022

51027261R00029